Maximize Your Self-Discipline

Brian E. Birchmeier, CHt

DEDICATION

I was adopted and for that I am forever grateful to my biological parents and to my Mom and Dad.

This work is dedicated to my MOM and DAD
Tom and Rita Birchmeier, I won the lottery of life when they chose me. Thanks!

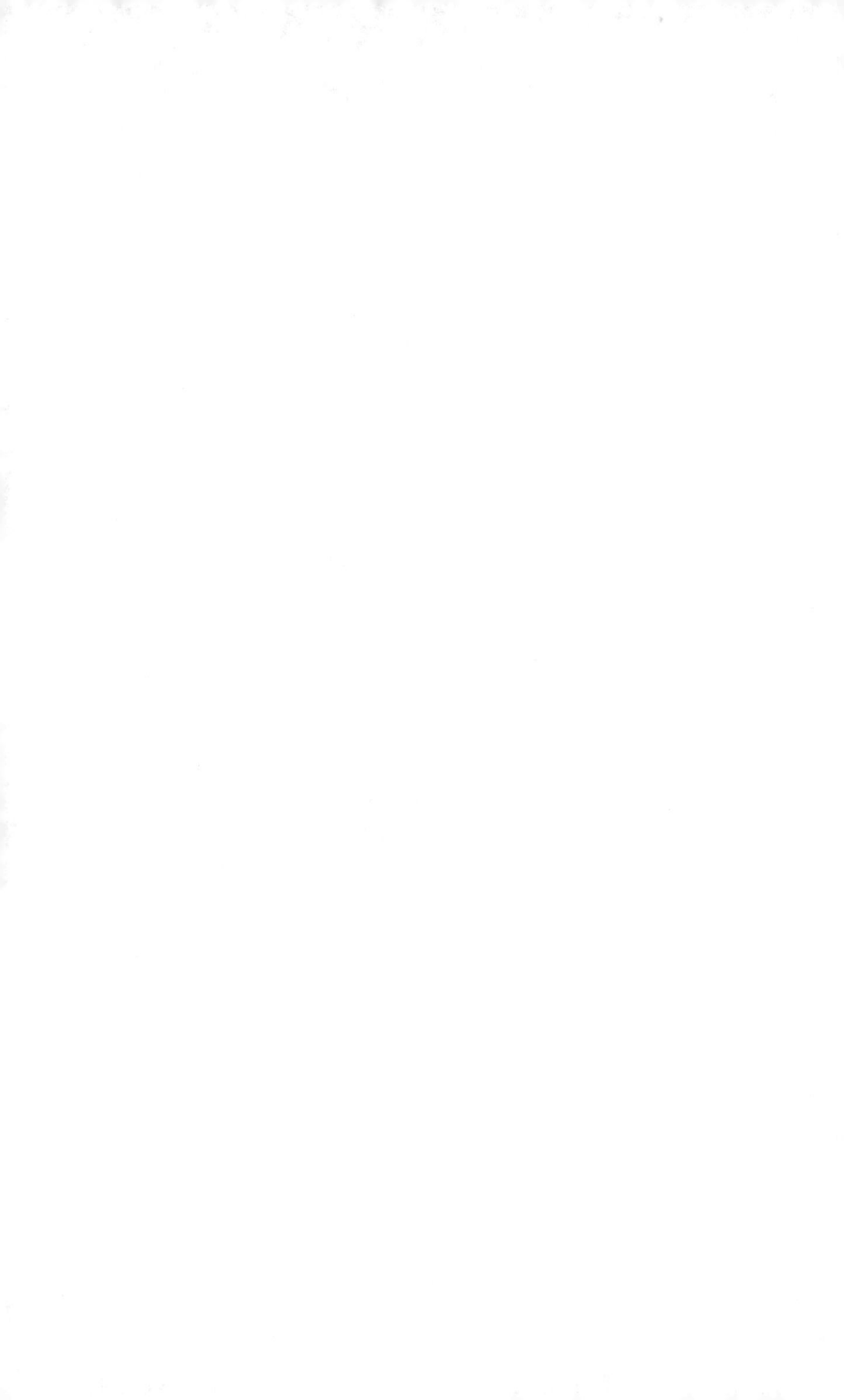

CONTENTS

ACKNOWLEDGMENTS

Feedback and critique are the foundation and cornerstone, respectively, for any work of this nature.

Our clients, readers, listeners and our advisors, too numerous to name without leaving very important people out, Thank you all. Without you we have no value.

1 CONCEPTS

In this chapter we will review the concepts used in creating this work and we will provide step by step instructions for you to create your own hypnotherapy and mindfulness sessions.

The Maximum Performance 4 x 4 Series provides effective and structured solutions to behavioral modification problems, ensuring that as long as you follow the steps, that your life is going to change.

The scripts included herein are made available with two groups in mind.

It is my hope that these will be used to guide professionals in helping to resolve their clients or patients issues.

I am also excited to see everyday people use these scripts as guides to create their own recordings. Recordings that can improve your life in any way that you decide appropriate.

If you are new to hypnosis, or if you have never recorded a hypnotherapeutic session for your own benefit I think that you are in for a pleasant surprise.

We've made the process easy and you may use this outline to prepare solutions to any issues that life may throw at you.

You may notice that the induction phase of the Foundation Session is quite long in relation to the other 4 hypnosis sessions. That is because one of the primary purposes of the Foundation Session is to introduce a deep state of hypnosis and then to anchor that state with a post hypnotic suggestion that states "The next time you listen to a hypnosis recording and it is safe to enter a very deep state of hypnosis, when you hear the words MPH Sleep Now you will go deeper into hypnosis than you have ever been before".

This phrase along with the other instructions allows you to use just one or two brief inductions, mention the phrase MPH Sleep Now and you are in. You've just saved 20 minutes of time for each subsequent recording. You may use the post hypnotic suggestion in your voice and it will have the same effect as if it were in mine.

In crafting your own sessions spend a brief period of time just allowing yourself to relax, engage the phrase "MPH Sleep Now – go deeper into hypnosis than you have ever been before" and then use any of the inductions that we have in this or any other process.

Once you have 3 to 5 minutes of an induction, ask the subconscious, and you may want to include spiritual guides consistent with your own beliefs and traditions, to use the processes learned in the Foundation Session to remove any issues or roadblocks that may be preventing you from reaching your goals. You may want to provide a minute or two of silence or music to allow time for these to work.

Your foundation is now set to work on anything. Go through each of the hypnotherapy sessions here and insert anything that you think may be helpful to your objective.

A few pointers that you should follow:

1. Be very clear as to what it is that you want to accomplish
2. Choose ONE (1) issue at a time to work on. For instance, if you want to quit smoking and to lose weight either record two separate sessions or combine them into a very clear objective of being lean, healthy and happy.
3. When choosing an objective, ask yourself what it is that attaining that goal will give you that you don't have now. Using the example from step 2 – what will 'freedom from smoking' and 'a lean body' give you that you don't have now.
4. List all of the reasons that you consciously want to change and then put them into your session. Always

leave room for your subconscious to add other reasons – there are always other reasons.

5. Make your statements in the present tense. Use phrases starting with "you are" rather than with "you will be"

6. Always state clearly and specifically the ideal you intend. For instance, you wouldn't say "Never think of a pink elephant again" – because as you read that, what did you think of? You wouldn't use the phrase "you are not fat anymore" because your subconscious does not respond to the qualifiers – all it sees is that you are fat. Instead use a phrase such as: "You are lean and healthy".

7. Put your recording on a device that is portable and easy to use. Most smart phones have the ability to download free audio recording apps – use one. Keep it simple and make it handy. There is an activation point in developing any new habit and the lower you can make all resistance the more likely it is for you to succeed.

8. Use your relaxing voice.

Here is an outline that you can follow. There is a copy of the outline and the pointers at www.maxphy.com on the FREE page.

Step 1: What do you want to accomplish with the recording?

Step 2: List all of the expectations that you have that once you achieve Step 1 that you will have that you don't have now.

Step 3: Determine the method of recording and assemble any equipment, apps, microphones, headsets, etc., which you may require.

Step 4: Outline your script – don't wing this. Have it written out and easy to read.

One Minute Relaxation – focus on your breathing, breathing in relaxation, breathing out tension

MPH Sleep Now and go deeper into hypnosis than you have ever been before

Insert the induction of your choice

Finish that induction with this: "and throughout this process the sound of my voice will continue to take you deeper and deeper into that wonderful state of therapeutic hypnosis, that state where changes that are important to you take place easily and effortlessly. The deeper you go the better you feel and the better you feel the deeper you go."

Ask your subconscious and spiritual guides to examine all of you throughout all time and space and locate anything that may be sabotaging your ability to achieve your objective. Use the instructions from the Foundation Session to resolve or remove any roadblocks to achieving the objective. Give yourself a minute or two to run through that process.

List all of the reasons that you want to accomplish this

objective. List your personal reasons; list the reasons that involve others. Be specific, be excited. Name them in the present tense as if they have already happened.

Give your subconscious and spiritual guides a minute or two to list additional reasons why accomplishing this objective is important.

Ask your spiritual guides and subconscious to provide you with healing dreams that will help to facilitate this process.

Ask your subconscious and spiritual guides to bring forward to your conscious mind any part of this process that is beneficial and life enhancing – but anything that the conscious mind is not yet ready to deal with, leave that behind until the appropriate time.

Restate the post hypnotic suggestion of "MPH Sleep Now".

Count out from one to five. I like to put a reinforcing statement after each number, such as 1 You are lean healthy and happy. 2 You are a wonderful example to your entire family., etc. Use statements that are important to you. Number 5 is always similar to – open your eyes feeling wonderful in every way.

If you have questions about designing your own processes you may reach us at results@maxphy.com, on Facebook at facebook.com/maxphy or at our website www.maxphy.com.

A few words are in order as to why combine Hypnotherapy and Mindfulness.

Hypnotherapy is the fastest way to bring about changes in the mind. Properly executed the processes included provide both permissions and framework for the subconscious and the mind to make correct the inner conflicts that sabotage our ability to succeed.

"It's all mental, I don't need hypnosis", has to be one of the funniest statements I've ever heard and it ironically makes my point very well.

Hypnosis is a naturally occurring state of mind. Young children exhibit signs of a hypnotic state through much of their waking hours until the age of about 4 years. Daydreaming, drifting off into worlds of thought, opening the door to both inner and outer awareness at the same time.

Over time those skills are used less and less as we mature.

Redeveloping these natural skills to allow ourselves to quickly resolve problems only makes sense.

Mindfulness Meditation has become a wonderful answer to so many issues. As I read I continue to see more and more references to this process. The sources seemed credible but even academia can get caught up in fads and trends.

The idea that focused attention could double nearly every therapy just seemed too much like hocus pocus to me. I realize the irony of reading that from a hypnotherapist.

The results of studies from the most prominent universities in the world were so consistent, so well done they were almost boring. Add 20 to 40 minutes of mindfulness meditation to the therapy and double the results.

There are few things in medicine, in science, that you can point to that will double the efficacy of the process – yet here we are implementing these practices that are thousands of years old.

I had used anchors, visualization and hypnosis for years with my athletes and business coaching clients so the natural question was, could Mindfulness Meditation impact their performance as suggested in the studies?

My experience is that there is no situation where being totally in the moment, accepting the moment for what it is and being aware of that present experience is not an improvement.

It is an improvement of performance as well as an improvement in the satisfaction of the event itself.

These audiobooks, from which the scripts for the sessions comprise the balance of these books combine the best practices of live sessions in formats that translate well to audio recordings.

There is no audio recording that can replace the skills of a highly trained, experienced hypnotherapist, but these come very close.

A note to hypnotists or hypnotherapists that may use these in their practice: We use ideomotor signals in all of our sessions. We don't have the client speak while hypnotized and that greatly reduces abreactions.

If you are not trained in using ideomotor signals or in aggressively seeking out impediments of all kinds, including, but not limited to, ego states, attachments, past lives – whatever format in which they may appear – get certified from a highly qualified school of hypnotherapy before using these processes.

This book will present the scripts found in the four audiobooks 'Elite Sales Success', Maximize Your Emotional Intelligence', 'Freedom From Distress and Anxiety' and '10 Supplemental Mindfulness Meditations'. The scripts for each will appear in this order.

You'll find that at times I digress from the scripts during the recordings. These are not transcripts, they are guides.

There are no magic words used here. Merlin would be bored.

These are, however, tried and true systems and processes that can provide measurable results for you and your clients if you follow the steps.

The Maximum Performance 4 x 4 Series provide effective and structured solutions to behavioral modification problems, ensuring that as long as you follow the steps of each program, that your life is going to change.

This is our mission.

Our core values are: Honesty, Humility, Hungry and Smart.

Together these create our culture.

Enjoy.

Have fun and get ready: Your Life Is About To Change!

2 INTRODUCTION & INSTRUCTIONS TO THE AUDIOBOOK

This chapter is your introduction and your Instructions for Maximize Your Self Discipline.

This program is not designed as a medical reference and is not intended to replace, diagnose or treat medical conditions or illness. If you have medical questions please direct them to your physician. If you are under the care of a physician or psychologist have them review this program before you begin.

Throughout this program you will be listening to and using hypnotherapeutic and meditative recordings. These are very powerful and they will affect your outer awareness, you may not listen to any of the sessions while operating any kind of machinery and certainly no driving.

These sessions will help you to establish new set points for your elevated levels of self-discipline, you will remove the roadblocks, those things inside of you that have been sabotaging your self-discipline in the past and you will set anchors that will ensure that your self-discipline has a safety net.

You may find all of our titles on Audible.com and iTunes.

Self-Discipline is one of the most widely sought out skills that we humans seek.

Self-Discipline is an essential skill in all areas of our life – it is also a very misunderstood part of our lives.

The fascinating aspect of self-discipline is that we all have it – every one of us, regardless of our mental acuity, our athletic ability, our business acumen or our social charms – we all have it and we all lack it.

I've had the pleasure of coaching, training and competing with many of the greatest strength athletes in the world of powerlifting. These remarkable men and women employ tremendous discipline to their training, their diets, their surroundings, their equipment. When they are in a cycle of training, bringing their strength to a peak at just the right time without injury – or at least attempting to keep injuries to a minimum – they are locked in, focused. They are at the gym early, they are staying late, they are studying video of every workout, they are perfecting flaws that only they and their coaches can see.

In the middle of their training cycle, however, ask them how they are doing on their finances? Ask them how they are doing on their relationships? Ask them how their job is going. Ask them how their maintenance of their home or their car is.

These hyper focused, highly self-disciplined athletes will tell you that they just have no self-discipline when it comes to those things.

Really?

If you bought this program I have to believe that you find yourself deficient in self-discipline in some area.

If you are like many of the elite people with whom we have worked in the business world, athletics, sales – you have areas of your life in which you exhibit strong self-discipline, don't you?

Of course you do, we all do. This program is going to help you improve your self-discipline skills, automatically!

If you have used our other 4 x 4 programs you'll be familiar with the format – this is designed to be an 8 week program.

You will combine hypnotherapeutic and mindfulness meditations to listen to.

Your Mindfulness practice will soon expand from our guided meditations – we love the fact that you are using these to establish your foundation, but it isn't about us – its about you and we haven't done our jobs until you are able to bring your attention to your present experience with acceptance at will.

It will begin with only a few moments of mindfulness – that is normal. As you practice, as with all things, you will gradually be able to extend your concentration for longer and longer periods of time.

As you progress through the guided meditations practice at every opportunity bringing your attention to the present moment with acceptance – that is, by the way, the definition of Mindfulness Meditation.

A few notes on practice: Perfect Practice makes Perfect, everything else perfects an error – that is paraphrased from the books of Harvey MacKay and he uses it throughout his works.

I like the term 'dedicated practice' as employed by Geoff Colvin in his book 'Talent is Overrated'. Dedicated practice acknowledges the fact that regardless of our efforts we are not perfect and we will never be.

Dedicated practice is the process of executing the activity, evaluating the activity and the results, correcting flaws, implementing the corrections and beginning the process again.

Why not concentrate only on the results? I mean, if you did this and you achieved that, and that is what you had hoped for or that was your goal, then, Yahoo – success, right?

Maybe!

If you used our other 4 x 4 programs you've heard me refer to humility. I define Humility in this as being aware that correlation does not necessarily mean causation.

How do you know that when you did this it was the cause of that? Perhaps That was going to happen anyway?

Look with a critical, yet compassionate eye at all parts of your practice. Make corrections, get 3rd party feedback, and implement the corrections, T.A.M.E. your practice, with compassion.

T.A.M.E stands for Test And Measure Everything.

So why does this process work?

The scientific term is experience dependent neuro plasticity – or in other words – the brain that fires together wires together.

Your brain is an amazing creation. It has the ability to adapt to your environment by creating new connections, new pathways and it will discard or in other words, disconnect, the pathways that it no longer requires.

It's like a railroad track with various switches along its path. As long as all of the switches remain the same every single train that follows in that direction will go to exactly the same place, they have to follow the tracks.

Now, throw a switch connecting two different tracks and every train that follows will have to go in the new direction, won't they?

Further imagine that some strange substance dissolves the switch and the old track, the old destination. After that happens no train will ever be able to go in exactly the old path ever again, will it?

That is the definition of changing behavior – changing the pathways so that you react differently to stimuli than you did before.

That's what you really want, isn't it?

You don't want to be in a situation where you have to think: "What was it that Brian said in chapter 3H?" Of course not – you want your brain, your mind, your body to react to the stimuli with self-discipline, automatically.

So lets get started.

This program is designed to last for 8 weeks – of course you may make it longer or shorter to fit your needs.

The reason for a program of this duration is that most research studies on activities like this indicate that over 8 weeks there are measurable and statistically significant results – you want measurable and statistically significant results.

I cue up a hypnotherapy recording on my phone and each morning after I wake I pop the headphones on and start my day. I then listen to a Mindfulness meditation or I'll meditate in a self-directed meditation for about 30 minutes.

These practices are very important to me and so I make sure that I make time, every day, for them.

In the context of this program, I would listen to a combination of hypnotherapy and mindfulness meditation, rotating every day. So say Monday, I'd listen to 1H and 1M, Tuesday 2H and 2M, Wednesday 3H and 3M and Thursday 4H and 4M. Friday I'd start over at 1H and 1M.

I only practice these on days that I breathe.

You may, of course, modify these to fit your life –

Remember Dedicated Practice: Make your plan –
Implement Your Plan, Determine corrections, Implement
corrections, and execute your plan!

A few other notes:

We determined as we developed these programs that
meditation positions was simply too exhaustive to include
without distracting from the processes themselves - There
are wonderful tutorials on line for innumerous and varied
meditation postures – please use them experiment with
different postures, expressions, mechanics. Make the
changes that you experience as you implement them the
objects of your awareness.

From a basic standpoint – you may be seated in a dignified
posture, as if a string were tied to the top of your head,
your body fully supported and mechanically sound.

You may also be lying down. I've never had trouble with
sleep when I meditate but I know that some people do.
Some disciplines suggest meditating at the top of a cliff or in
other precarious situations – I'll leave that one to you.

Mindfulness Meditation is defined as being aware of your
present experience with acceptance.

Nowhere in that definition does it say that you are going to
be relaxed. There may be times that you are relaxed and
there may be times when the experience is very intense.

How about the term acceptance?

Acceptance in this context does not mean that you don't need to or want to change something. It does not mean that you have to settle for anything.

Acceptance in this context means that you are being true to yourself and all others with exactly where you are.

Acceptance in this concept refers to a lack of deception of both yourself and others.

Acceptance means that you have an accurate starting point increasing the likelihood of your ending up where you want.

I've talked mostly about Mindfulness so far but you may be curious about the hypnotherapeutic portions of the program.

I use the term hypnotherapeutic because these processes are designed to actively change anything that may be inhibiting the changes that you are seeking. In all of the hypnosis recordings that I've been able to find the process is simple – there is an induction taking you into a state of hypnosis and then there are positive affirmations.

These are wonderful for relaxing but they tend to have limited efficacy unless there are no internal conflicts.

You know those crazy conversations, arguments and fights you have with yourself?

Yup, those.

This process aligns those parts of you that are arguing so that if both sides of the argument have your best interests in mind, that they come together to ensure that you achieve the self-discipline that you require. If these arguments do not have your best interests in mind they are removed so that they never impede your self-discipline ever again.

You will not be going to sleep during these processes – hypnosis is very different than sleep. You will still be aware of your surroundings but through these processes your inner awareness opens up and in this state remarkable change that is important to you takes place.

You can't be made to do something that you do not already want to do – regardless of the stuff you see on TV or in the movies.

Your mind may use all of your senses in displaying whatever it is that you need to experience in order to identify issues and to implement resolutions.

In this way your state will resemble a dream in that your experiences may have nothing to do with reality.

Just because you dream of a fire breathing dragon or experience one in hypnosis, doesn't mean that you'll have singed toes.

You may see yourself in ancient times, or on a spaceship, even as other people or different genders.

I don't get caught up in the arguments of these being real or not – it can't and won't be proven either way and for the purposes of maximizing your self-disciple, that argument is irrelevant.

My concern is that we locate the issues sabotaging your self-discipline, we resolve or remove those impediments and we achieve the results that you hoped for when you purchased this program.

This will be an amazing experience for you. Enjoy this process.

Begin with the Foundation Session – that will provide the cues and post hypnotic suggestions that all of the following sessions require enabling them to be much more brief and effective than they otherwise would need to be.

After that – follow your plan, make changes as you find them necessary, implement them and enjoy the process to Maximize Your Self-Discipline.

3 THE FOUNDATION SESSION

This initial recording will set the foundation for all of the hypnotherapy recordings to come. It contains specific instructions to the subconscious allowing the subsequent recordings to be much less extensive than they otherwise would need to be.

If you've used other 4 x 4 Series from us – first of all, Thank YOU! You do not need to listen to this foundational recording again unless you feel the need for a refresher. We keep all of the signals and post hypnotic suggestions the same from one 4 x 4 program to the next so that each reinforces the others.

So find a safe place where you can begin your hypnotic journey. Make yourself comfortable, you may be seated or lying down. Uncross your arms and your legs and begin to notice your breath.

This process is very powerful and even if you intend to listen only casually, it will affect your outer awareness. Do not listen to this recording while operating any kind of machinery or automobile; listening while driving is absolutely prohibited.

Allow your body to move as it feels the need during this process; if you have to wiggle then wiggle. It is not unusual for emotions and feelings find a particular body part in which to make you aware. Just note the body part until later and perhaps bring that to your attention in an upcoming hypnosis or meditation session.

Now, just focus on your breathing, breathing in relaxation, breathing out tension.

Progressive induction head to toe

Eye closure 3 times

Light and Mist in the Morning

10 Stairs breathing in bringing the door closer and out opening it a little bit more – safe place

If you feel comfortable with your spiritual side, welcome your friends or family, spiritual guides or teachers, guardian angels or religious figures who may be with you to help guide and protect you through these processes. Allow them to come in at any point and assist with keeping you safe and bringing about the solutions and resolutions that you enact; have them lock any positive and life enhancing changes into place so that they continue to be a force that compels you to be the calm, happy confident person that you truly are.

As your conscious mind rests in that wonderful safe place, Subconscious, go through these processes as many times as is required. Continue this work even when not in a state of hypnosis and modify and perfect it for you based on your own beliefs and traditions.

As you review your entire existence through all time and space, determine in descending order – from the most influential to least – any experience outside influence whose actions are standing in the way, are sabotaging your *Maximum your Self Discipline*.

As you deal with the experience and the defense mechanism or response that was developed from that experience – determine the purpose of the reaction or habit: was it meant to keep you safe, to protect you from harm in the future or is it punishing you or otherwise attempting to cause distress in your life?

Determine if the decisions that stem from this experience are intended to be in your best interests and if they are intended to be in your best interests but are no longer enhancing your life, be aware that the reaction is causing harm & offer for that experience to once again be a part of the whole you that is working together to Reveal the *Disciplined* YOU!

Let the experience know that they no longer have to fight and struggle all alone – knowing that their efforts have been futile and in fact are hurting you, the person they most want to help. Free them from any emotions of baggage associated with the experience. As soon as the old role is permanently released so that it never ever is able to bother you or anyone else ever again, then select a new role, acceptable to all, one that is more powerful, that is life enhancing and one that guarantees your Maximum Self Discipline.

Imagine for a minute how easy it will be for you to

Maximize your **Self Discipline** with all parts of you aligned to the same goal – to the same commitment.

This is the real you!

Take a few moments to review all of your existence, through all time and space and align or remove anything that is impeding your maximum self discipline.

60

Occasionally there will something that just simply won't relinquish their destructive role and when that happens wrap them in a snug blanket of light so that their influence cannot hurt you or anyone else ever again. Bring in any assistance you may need to permanently remove these issues from ever causing you harm ever again.

Often these will hide and by their nature they are deceptive. Be patient and vigilant. When you see or feel their influence request all of the help you require, protect yourself with the light and remove them – you do this easily and effortlessly even when you are not in a state of hypnosis.

You notice that each day that you become more aligned, more unified and stronger. The focus on being healthy makes the choices easier to make, the training easier and more enjoyable and the temptations less and less. Your results are tremendous; you enjoy Maximizing your **Self Discipline**.

Feel the power growing within you, the confidence, and the joy.

This is the real you.

Take a few moments to review all parts of your existence and align or remove anything that has been standing in the way of your Maximum Self Discipline.

60

It's now time to take you now on a journey – to show you your life 10 years from now.

Today, this moment, you freed yourself and revealed the real YOU!

You are Free from the delusions and illusions that kept you from being the real you.

Notice how you feel? Feel the satisfaction of knowing that this is the real you. Notice all of the other emotions that are associated with your new lifestyle.

As you see yourself along the timeline from today and forward the next 10 years see all of the wonders of your world that your Maximum Self Discipline make real.

See how every day builds on the former and provides a foundation for the next so that your amazing self-discipline continues to grow and grow.

Feel the love that others have for you – and that you have

for you.

Feel the gratitude that you have for enjoying **Maximum Self Discipline**.

Experience the leader that is you.

Notice how your family sees you. See the impact that your Calm, healthy, humble, **disciplined** and happy lifestyle has on each of them. See the influence that you've had – see the positive choices that they have made because of your influence.

Enjoy the humility that comes with seeing the negative choices that they have avoided because of your influence.

Feel the satisfaction of having the means to support organizations and people that do amazing things. You make the world a better place every single day.

The skills and talents that you have developed and exposed in the process of discovering the real you – calm, confidence*, **discipline***, health, happiness and serenity have become skills that you've been able to pass along to others. The Elite Person that you are provides tremendous benefits to you and to all you influence.

Now magnify these wonderful feelings. Make them twice as strong, now three times until they are nearly overwhelming.

Now absorb these wonderful feelings into every atom, every molecule that is your body, that is your being – for this is the real you, You have Revealed the **Disciplined**

Person that is YOU and you produce consistently superior results; you are comfortable in knowing that you deserve it.

Each day the subconscious will find 10, 15, 20 perhaps more things that delight you – that make you happy. Perhaps a sunrise, a flower, an act of kindness – it can be anything. Notice how happy it makes you – notice the joy that it gives you and then multiply it just like we did before – make it 2 3 perhaps more times as intense and then absorb those feelings into every atom, every molecule that is your body.

When something unpleasant occurs link that unpleasantness with the next event – continue to do so until it has no negative effects on you.

Events that used to ruin your day or your experience are forever gone because it will quickly and easily be absorbed into and by the wonderful feelings that you've absorbed into every molecule of the mist that is your body.

The next time that you listen to a Hypnotherapeutic recording and it is safe to enter a very deep state of therapeutic hypnosis you'll hear me say the words **MPH Sleep Now** and you'll instantly and effortlessly go even more deeply into that wonderful state of hypnosis than you've ever been.

I ask the subconscious to provide you with healing dreams – dreams that continue the process of the **Maximum Self Discipline** that is YOU!

Subconscious to bring forward to your conscious mind any

helpful life enhancing aspects of this session, but to leave behind anything that the conscious mind is not yet ready to deal with until the appropriate time.

If it is time to sleep when this session is over then you will ignore the instructions to return to outer awareness and as I count from 1 to 5 you will easily transition into a deep healing sleep awakening refreshed and energetic, confident, disciplined and serene.

If you do awaken when you prefer to be asleep, or if at any time you need assistance getting to sleep, all you ever need to do is to take three deep breaths and then breathing normally count from 10 down to 1 and well before you reach the end you'll have fallen deeply into a deep healing restful sleep.

And now if it is time to return to return to outer awareness. I will count from 1 to 5 and when I reach 5 you will awaken wonderfully refreshed, energetic, balanced and centered and ready for your day.

1 You have Maximum Self Discipline

2 Your mind and body are more aligned, determined and focused than ever before

3 You can feel the anticipation and energy growing inside of you

4 Smile – you are on your way and

5 open your eyes feeling wonderfully refreshed, balanced,

centered, energetic, disciplined and enthusiastic, ready for your day.

4 REMOVING ROADBLOCKS - HYPNOTHERAPY

Roadblocks are anything that keeps you from accomplishing your goals.

In relation to Self-Discipline that becomes an interesting challenge because a lack of discipline is likely to be the reason why you invested in this program.

Use food as an example – say that you were raised to fill your plate, take a bit of everything available and that it was required that you eat everything – even if it meant sitting at the table long after everyone else had left until you could finally choke down the last few bites. This experience probably stayed with you for a while, agreed?

Perhaps when you were a bit older you were praised for being such a 'good eater' and the praise was enough for you to take more than you really wanted in order to live up to your reputation. Or to earn more praise.

Perhaps more recently, body weight and composition, health concerns and appearance come into play and you've decided to lose some fat. You've educated yourself, you have a decent understanding of what your body needs to be healthy and you have a game plan for diet and exercise.

Think about the conversations in your mind between the experiences of eating everything on your plate no matter what, the reputation for eating large amounts of food and your new knowledge of the quantity and quality you require to meet your goals – see a conflict here?.

Imagine that you have a good week into your diet and exercise program when you have to be at a function at a buffet. You've made good progress and with a sterile environment that you created around your home – you dumped all of the junk food - your Nutritionally Aware self has been in control with little impact from the others.

Now you are handed a heaping plate filled with food. Your nutritionally aware self looks at everything on the plate looking for anything that is beneficial to your body.

You begin eating and now you are at the point where in the sterile environment you would be satiated – you've consumed all of the nutrition your body needs.

But then the self that was trained to finish every last bite regardless of anything else kicks in and is screaming to clean the plate.

Oh, and here comes the self that takes great pride in eating more than anyone else and it has something to say.

What do you think the likelihood is that you will stop eating at the satiation point? Do you think that line might get blurred a little?

You can apply this scenario with its own unique casts of characters to anything from waking earlier to cleaning out your inbox for emails.

There are parts of you that are convinced that it is in your best interests to avoid that which you would call Self Discipline.

The process of removing roadblocks aligns the various conflicting events, emotions, inclinations, selves – you may call them what you will – to align each to compel you to be self-disciplined.

I like the example of playing tug-o-war and as the alignment progresses the members of the opposing side drop their rope and run to your side to pull – before long there is no-one on the other side and there is no option other than Maximum Self Discipline.

So with that in mind, take some time and find a safe place to go into a very deep state of therapeutic hypnosis – that state where changes that are important to you take place easily and effortlessly.

15

Please do not listen to this recording while operating machinery of any kind; of course driving while listening is prohibited. This will affect your outer awareness; it is very powerful so even if you intend to listen casually, Do Not Listen and Drive!

15

Focus on your breathing, feeling yourself relax and melting

into a wonderful state of therapeutic hypnosis, notice that you are breathing in relaxation and out tension with every breath.

Every breath takes you deeper and deeper, more and more relaxed.

As we begin this process we'll be searching for anything that may be objecting to your having Maximum Self Discipline.

Your subconscious will follow the instructions from the Foundational Hypnotherapy recording to resolve the issues.

MPH Sleep Now – go deeper into hypnosis than you have ever been before.

See as you go deeper and deeper that all of those feelings or voices that used to help convince you to settle for less than being Elite – see that they have all taken on new roles. Roles that are stronger and more powerful than ever they were before – and these new roles exist to ensure that you are Elite – you are compelled to succeed!

See yourself walking along a wonderful sandy shore. Notice that your breath is easy and effortless. Your body already knows how to breathe. Notice that each time you go through a cycle of breathing in and out you go deeper and deeper into the therapeutic realm of hypnosis where wonderful changes take place easily and effortlessly.

As you walk along this sandy shore notice as you look up that a series of light fluffy clouds are floating past and as you notice each one you become twice as relaxed, twice as deep, deeper and deeper.

You find yourself counting these light fluffy clouds backwards from 10 down to 1 and each time you count you are twice as deep as you were before. 10, 9 8 7 6 5 4 3 2 1

And as you reach the last cloud you notice that you've arrived at a wonderful safe place and just allow your conscious mind to go to that safe place and let it do whatever it needs to do. Your subconscious mind will take care of everything for you. Sometimes your conscious mind will be paying attention and sometimes not but your subconscious mind will hear everything.

Subconscious, we are embarking on a journey to uncover the Maximum Self Discipline that has always been here. Please examine every part of your existence and locate each and every event that is standing in the way, sabotaging the process of allowing your Maximum Self-Discipline to prevail..

Locate each one starting with the most powerful first and resolve each one step by step including assigning any new roles that will make them champions for your Maximum Self-Discipline.

Bring in any assistance consistent with your beliefs and traditions.

This process will go very quickly and if it is not completed as the recording proceeds, continue until finished and all issues are resolved, new roles assigned and uncooperative aspects safely removed so that they will never bother you or anyone else every again.

2 minutes of background music

Subconscious, if you are continuing to work with issues, please continue and complete your mission.

Once complete I'd like for you to guide a tour of what it means to have *Amazing Self Discipline*.

See yourself 10 years from now.

You are able to make the changes internally very quickly. You came to realize that these well-intentioned but misguided 'selves' needed to have new roles or had to be neutralized and you practiced this process until everyone was pulling on your side of the rope

Things that used to stop you or get in the way no longer have any impact on you. You have *Amazing Self Discipline.*

You are calm and collected making rational decisions in real time easily and effortlessly.

You are free!

Whenever something presents itself that requires you to exercise your Maximum Self-Discipline you integrate it easily and effortlessly into your daily activities.

You make your decisions after careful deliberation –

considering all aspects and then you set it aside once the decision is make so that you are free to focus on life.

You have an amazing intuition.

You only participate in emotions or activities which are likely to have a positive impact on the situation.

Every day you perfect the systems and processes that contribute to your *Amazing Self Discipline*.

You empower those around you so that your life runs just as well with you not there as it does when you are hands on. Your freedom contributes to your *self-discipline*.

Your family life and close friends – all of your relationships are greatly improved and as you have felt better about yourself and gained wonderful insight and perspective.

Just like a pebble tossed into a still pond, your circles of influence extend out thousands of times greater than the pebble itself.

You appreciate the humility of knowing that you've been able to help so many other people.

You enjoy the happiness of knowing the impact you've had on your friends and family's lives.

Allow those emotions to grow and swell – magnify those wonderful emotions until they are nearly overwhelming and then absorb them into every atom, every molecule that is your body. Knowing that this is the real you.

Go out 20 years. Notice the life that you are able to lead and how your **Amazing Self Discipline** has contributed to it.

See how people treat you.

Notice how people are drawn to your happiness – your personality has become magnetic and you attract many interesting people.

See the positive influence that you've had on your family and friends – and how that positive influence has magnified. The world is so much better for you having been here.

See the wonderful decisions that people have made because of your positive influence – what great feelings.

See the poor decisions that were NOT made because of your influence – what tremendous gratitude.

Magnify these feelings and absorb them into ever molecule that is the mist that is your body – this is the real you! All of the rest was just an illusion.

Each day you will consciously or subconsciously notice 15 or 20 or more things that make you happy – and each time you will magnify that happy feeling to the point that it is nearly overwhelming, and you'll absorb it into every part of your body and soul – and you'll notice that each day you feel happier, brighter – like nothing can get you down.

The next time that you listen to one of these recordings and it is safe for you to enter into hypnosis, when you hear me say **MPH Sleep Now** you'll instantly and effortlessly go deeper into hypnosis than you have ever been before.

I ask your subconscious to bring forward to your conscious mind anything from this process that is helpful and life enhancing but any memories that may be harmful – leave them behind to be dealt with at the appropriate time.

If it is time for you to sleep you will ignore the instructions to return to outer awareness and instead, will transition into a deep state of restful, healing REM sleep, awakening on time and completely refreshed.

And now it's time to return to outer awareness. I'll count from 1 to 5 and when I reach 5 you'll open your eyes feeling wonderfully refreshed, balanced, centered in every way.

1. You have *Amazing Self Discipline*
2. You know that you will always be calm happy and serene
3. You empower all around you to be better
4. Smile you are almost there and
5. Open your eyes feeling wonderful in every way

5 THE BREATH AWARENESS MEDITIATON

Breath Awareness is a fundamental building block that can be employed with any situation to help you bring your attention to the present moment. We use this in every guided meditation in our program.

The purpose of the breath awareness meditation is to help you develop your skill of concentration.

Mindfulness is about being aware of your present experience with acceptance, no past, no future – just this moment.

Throughout your days whenever you find your mind wandering or restless, just bring your attention back to your breath, making it the object of your awareness.

Situational awareness is essential to **self-discipline** – it allows you to pick up signals from the world around you. As you develop your concentration you'll find yourself relating to the rest of the world far differently.

use the breath meditation as a staring place for self-directed meditations at any time and place, allowing you to fix attention on the immediate present surroundings; placing you totally in the moment with only the moment as it exits.

This meditation works best with your eyes closed, but if you find yourself drifting off to sleep, feel free to open your eyes, gently bringing your attention back to the present. Some disciplines suggest meditating at the top of a cliff or the edge of a well to keep your mind alert. Meditation is about awareness, not necessarily relaxation.

This will affect your outer awareness and you are not allowed to listen to this recording while operating machinery of any kind – certainly no driving.

If you haven't already done so, find a posture that is comfortable for you, Notice your breath – you may notice it at the tip of your nose, the cooler air flowing in and the warmer air flowing out. Perhaps you notice it more in your mouth or maybe you are breathing with your belly and notice the sensations there.

30:

As you practice – bring your attention to the different parts of your body and find what works best for you. See where you are most aware of your breath.

30:

Follow through full cycles of breathing in and breathing out.

30:

Notice any thoughts that may come into your consciousness – just allow them to be there and pass of their own accord, no pushing or shoving. If you drift away just gently bring your attention back to your breath.

30:

If you find that your mind is playing storyteller – a job that it is very good at – just gently bring your awareness back to your breath.

30:

If you find your mind wandering you may want to experiment with labeling your breaths in and out. Stay focused on each breath and use the label to direct your attention to the breath.

30:

You may also count your breaths but limit the count to any two numbers. 1 and 2, or 47 and 47. Don't allow the counting to progress. Just repeat the numbers, using them to direct your attention back to your breath.

30:

From time to time you'll notices feelings or sensations in the body, maybe an itch, maybe a cramp or an ache – try not to react to it. Bring your attention to the physical sensation and just be with it. Notice all of the different aspects to the sensation – if it is very uncomfortable feel free to move

30:

Notice how each breath is different from the others. Be curious compare your breaths with each other

30:

As you develop more concentration allow your breathing to take place naturally – your body knows how to breathe and what it needs – just let it happen – accept what your body is doing.

30:

If you notice that your thoughts judgmental – perhaps thinking how well you are doing, or how poorly, that you like or dislike what you are doing – just allow them to pass – bring your attention back to your breath.

30:

Be just in this moment and at this moment there is nothing else – nowhere else to be. Practice awareness and acceptance of each moment.

30:

All is perfect, just the way it is, including your desire to change and improve. Welcome the various stimuli as opportunities to fully experience the sensations

30:

Know that you cannot fail at this practice

30:

Is your concentration better at the beginning, middle or end of this session?

30:

Bring your concentration back to your breath

30:

As you have some concentration – bring to mind the idea of Maximum Self Discipline and make that meaning the object of your awareness

(note to return to this subject as the object of awareness every 60 seconds until the end)

Well Done

6 LOWER YOUR ACTIVATION POINTS - HYPNOTHERAPY

We all have self-discipline for the things that we have to do every day. Sometimes that self-discipline just needs to be re-directed until the new habits that you are creating take over and become a part of your everyday activities.

Your Activation Point is the amount of energy required to affect a change from the path of least resistance.

For instance, watching TV has been proven in study after study to be less rewarding and leads people to be less happy than 'hands on hobbies', and yet on average Americans watch over 5 hours of television each day – that takes amazing self-discipline – do you realize how much dedication, training, discipline and effort it took to get to a point where you could sit in front of an electronic device for 5 hours a day, more than 35 hours each week 365 days a year? One thousand eight hundred and twenty five hours per year, wow! That is more than enough hours to qualify for a full time job!

The small amount of effort required to use remote controls, DVR's, On Demand and streaming services dramatically impacts our ability to bring our attention away from watching TV toward the other things that we want to do or accomplish – even when we know that the other things are more enjoyable.

Take aware remote controls and TV hours drop like a rock.

Perhaps another way of describing it may be that the activation point of an activity is essentially the level of difficulty beyond which we are either willing or unwilling to proceed.

Let's use one of my challenges: If peanut butter is in the house that is my weak point when losing weight – I am more likely to give into a craving than if the peanut butter is at the store; I probably won't drive to buy a jar to satisfy an evening craving.

We can lower our activation point in several ways – we can sleep in our workout clothes if we are trying to develop a habit of training in the mornings, we can hide the remote controls so that we have to get up to change the channels, we can get rid of the junk food in our house so that we have to leave in order to have a food binge, we can modify our phones and computers so that we are not distracted from our primary tasks and duties, we can set rules for ourselves so that we avoid making simple yet destructive choices. These are all conscious methods of changing activation points

This process is going to give you a boost so that you automatically, unconsciously modify the activation points, allowing you to Maximize Your Self-Discipline.

Webster's Dictionary defines self-discipline as: the ability to make yourself do things that should be done.

So let's get ready and excited to lower the activation point for Maximizing Your Self Discipline.

Please do not listen to this recording while operating machinery of any kind; obviously, driving while listening is prohibited.

Find a comfortable place to enter hypnosis. You may be lying down or seated. You may find it helpful to leave your legs and arms uncrossed; above all, be comfortable.

And as you focus on your breathing, feeling yourself relax and melting into a wonderful state of therapeutic hypnosis, notice that you are breathing in relaxation and out tension with every breath.

Every breath takes you deeper and deeper, more and more relaxed. ***MPH Sleep Now*** – go deeper into hypnosis than you have ever been before.

Notice a wonderful feeling of relaxation above your head and feel as it washes slowly over you like a warm welcome soft breeze. As it reaches your forehead it relaxes ever muscle, every bit of tension located in your forehead and scalp. Feel it as it flows over your cheeks – relaxing every muscle around your eyes, relaxing your jaw – all the tension that you often store in your jaw just melts away – easily and effortlessly.

The relaxation flows over your neck to your shoulders – instantly removing any tension stored there – relaxing everything from front to back, side to side, easily and effortlessly. Notice the relaxation flowing over your chest and abdomen relaxing all of the muscles from front to back, side to side – all of the muscles of your back – large and small – completely relax leaving your body fully supported and care free. You notice that your body is just a perfect temperature, not too hot, not too cold, perfectly balanced and centered.

The relaxation flows over your hips relaxing the muscles of your hips, thighs moving to your lower legs and as the relaxation reaches your feet you feel peaceful and content, as if you just received a complete body massage. You feel safe, peaceful and relaxed.

Notice a spot on your forehead, just above your nose and at the level of your eyebrows – focus on that spot for a bit, I know that your eyes will be fatigued shortly but just focus on that spot and as you do, feel all of the muscles around your eyes just relax, relax to the point that it just feels pointless to open them. You can give them a try if you want, and you know that you could open them at any time that you needed to but it just seems like too much trouble.

30

As you continue to listen to the sound of my voice you realize that all along you have had all of the tools required to be able to do the things that need to be done – in other words, you already have Amazing Self Discipline, you just needed to learn the skills that allow that amazing self-discipline to be set free.

Your basic instincts are to take the path of least resistance, this stems from our ancient times when it was a matter of life and death to burn less energy than it took to consume energy. To not do that meant starvation.

Understanding this makes it easier to be compassionate towards yourself for times that you have not been disciplined – it also provides you with an additional tool to understand that when your mind and body object to your doing something they are acting instinctively to conserve energy.

You can be grateful for the instinct and yet consciously and subconsciously override it so that you are effective. There are lots of calories of energy to be consumed and you are in no danger of starving or operating at a deficit unless you choose to.

Knowing that your instinct is to take the path of least resistance you recognize situations in which you may encounter trouble and you make those situations easier to exercise your discipline by lowering the activation point – or the amount of energy required to do the disciplined activity rather than the passive one.

If you are developing a habit of training in the mornings but you would much rather sleep in – you may sleep in your workout clothes, knowing that the effort to get out of the clothes would be greater than getting up and getting going.

If you are developing the habit of returning phone calls or emails quickly and ensuring an empty in box you may set up rules for yourself that limits the amount of time a message can be there before it is acted upon.

If you are developing habits of reducing impulse purchases you may decide to leave your credit cards locked in a drawer at home or to reduce the amount of cash that you have with you at any given time.

If you are attempting to change your body weight or composition, creating a sterile environment – one that is free of the foods that you eat spontaneously that are not in your best interests makes it more difficult to splurge.

Take a few moments to review the areas of your life in which you want to develop Amazing Self Discipline and develop some strategies that you can enact right now to make it easy easy easy to make yourself do things that should be done.

2 minutes of music

Now see yourself doing all of the things that should be done.

Notice how much easier all of your life is now that this is your habit

Notice how other people follow your example

Notice how the lives of other people are improved because of the example that you set

See yourself continuing to improve over the next 10 years

This is the real you – you are ***amazingly self-disciplined*** and you enjoy being an effective person.

You continue to improve every day.

If it is time for you to sleep you will ignore the instructions to return to outer awareness and when I count from 1 to 5 you will transform from your state of hypnosis to a wonderful state of deep healing, restful REM sleep, awakening on time, refreshed, energetic with amazing self discipline.

If it is time to return to outer awareness when I count from 1 to 5 you will emerge from this wonderful state of hypnosis feeling tremendously refreshed, energetic with amazing self-discipline with compassion in your heart and a smile on your face.

1. You have Amazing Self Discipline
2. You get things done that need to be done
3. You are an wonderful example to all that you influence
4. Your Amazing Self Discipline makes everyone around you better and
5. Open your eyes feeling wonderful in every way

7 THE LOVING KINDNESS MEDITATION

The Loving Kindness Meditation is an integral part of many disciplines. It is widely accepted that in order to bring about change we must accept the situation as is – accepting means that you are not fighting it.

You may also hear it referred to as Meta.

Have you ever noticed that when you are trying to make a change that the more you fight it the more of a hold it has on you?

I had Chinese handcuffs as a child – and the harder I pulled my fingers apart the tighter they became – changing habits or mindsets is similar.

Accepting you as you are right now is fundamental. After all, believing anything different is to delude yourself – you would be starting with an error.

This above all: *to thine own self be true*, And it must follow, as the night the day, Thou canst not then be false to any man.

Shakespeare wrote these words 4 centuries ago, they still hold true. If you deceive yourself - you fail.

Be true to yourself and you will then be true and honest with all others.

The loving Kindness meditation develops your sense of

compassion – for yourself and others.

It is rare that I don't get objections from the tough men and women of the world over this one. For some reason it is believed that compassion means being soft. Or that they have been told that standing in front of a mirror telling lies to yourself and making believe that you are something you are not is obviously more productive than compassion.

Nothing could be further from the truth. Compassion for yourself and for others provides perspective, allows for wisdom and creates clarity.

Strength comes from accepting your present experience and fully being aware of it.

Loving Kindness practices may be applied to anything; yourself, your business, your team, your friends, your family, your community, your country or your world.

You'll employ some body mechanics in this exercise as well as throughout the course. Sometimes you'll bring a smile to your face – and notice the difference that you feel in your body; experiment with different kinds of smiles. We'll also place a hand over our heart and another over that hand – and again – notice the differences in sensations anywhere in your body. Notice as you practice how different postures or positions affect your experience.

It's important to know that there is no magic in these words and phrases. We use a wide variety and encourage you to use the phrases that mean something to you. During this process I'll repeat a phrase and then give you a few moments to focus on that phrase, repeating it to yourself or out loud as you wish – or you may use a phrase of your own.

So with that, assume your favorite meditation posture. This exercise involves visualizing so you may wish to be seated or lying down. This will affect your outer awareness so you may not listen to this while driving.

If you have not already begin to do so – start following your breath – through a full cycle, wherever you have the best sensations, could be the tip of your nose, or your mouth. It may be the expansion and contraction of your chest or the movement of your belly.

30:

As you develop concentration bring to mind someone or something that embodies unconditional love. It could be a religious figure or a family member. It could be someone you've read about or imagined, it could be a pet.

30:

Place your hand over your heart and then cover that with the other hand. As you extend your thoughts to that naturally loving being – extend the loving kindness to them – saying – May you be Happy, May you be peaceful, May you be free from Suffering.

30:

May you be Free, May you find peace, May you have grace and courage.

If you feel resistance just allow it to be there, bring your attention back to the phrases or to your breath

30

Imagine that loving being extending the same to you

May you be happy, May you be peaceful, May you be free from Suffering.

30:

Extend these wishes to yourself for a moment

May I be FREE, May I Find Peace, May I have Grace and Courage

30

Bring a slight, loving smile to your face: May I be safe, May I be loving, May I live in peace, May I be safe, May I be loving, May I live in peace

30:

May I be calm, May I be healthy, May I be happy, May I be calm, May I be healthy, May I be Happy

30:

Happy.....Peaceful.......Free; Safe............Loving.........Peace;

Calm.....Healthy........Happy x 2

30:

And now extend that Loving Kindness to a larger group of people, perhaps your family or friends

May you be happy, May you be Peaceful, May you be free from Suffering; May you be Safe, May you be Healthy, May you Live in Peace; May you be Calm, May you be Healthy, May you be Happy.... X 2

30:

And now extend Loving Kindness to your whole community

May you be free, may you find peace, may you have grace and courage

May you be happy, May you be Peaceful, May you be free from Suffering;

30:

And now extend Loving Kindness to your entire state or province:

May you be happy, May you be Peaceful, May you be free from Suffering; May you be Safe, May you be Healthy, May you Live in Peace; May you be Calm, May you be Healthy, May you be Happy.... X 2

30:

If you find it helps add the slight loving smile as you meditate

Now extend Loving Kindness to your entire country:

May you be happy, May you be Peaceful, May you be free from Suffering; May you be Safe, May you be Healthy, May you Live in Peace; May you be Calm, May you be Healthy, May you be Happy…. X 2

30:

And the entire world:

May you be free, may you find peace, may you have grace and courage.

30:

And to all parts of the universe that can benefit:

May you be happy, May you be Peaceful, May you be free from Suffering; May you be Safe, May you be Healthy, May you Live in Peace; May you be Calm, May you be Healthy, May you be Happy

30:

Continue by bringing this back to your self

May I be happy, May I be Peaceful, May I be free from Suffering; May I be Safe, May I be Healthy, May I Live in Peace; May I be Calm, May I be Healthy, May I be Happy…. X 2

30:

Bring to mind the reasons for beginning this program, the reasons why you want to Maximize your self-discipline.

30

Bring to mind an event in which you did not exercise self-discipline, and repeat to yourself

May you find peace, may you be free, may you have grace and courage.

30

Over the next few moments bring to mind instances when you did not exercise self-discipline

Use a phrase that allows for you to forgive yourself.

Keep in mind that forgiveness does not condone the offence – it merely frees you from it.

May you forgive, may you be forgiven, may you be free

May you be happy, May you be Peaceful, May you be free from Suffering;

From Me to you

May you be Safe, May you be Healthy, May you Live in Peace;

May you be Calm, May you be Healthy, May you be Happy.... X 2

Well Done

8 MAXIMUM MOTIVATION HYPNOTHERAPY

Ask a dozen people to define motivation and you will get a dozen different answers?

Motivation is defined by Webster's Dictionary as simply the desire to do things.

Often of the cause of so called 'un motivated people' is a lack of clarity as to what it is that they want to accomplish and why.

It may be conflicts of deep seated beliefs or paradigms.

'I want to be wealthy', conflicts with 'money is the root of all evil'.

'I want to be slim' conflicts with 'only narcissistic people are slim'.

Research Motivation and you'll get everything from goal

setting to affirmations – and most of the suggested activities appear to resemble a recipe for magic spells rather than a solid foundation for change.

So what is it – how do we get our self motivated – say the definition – how do we desire to do things?

Purpose, Clarity and Action.

If you are clear on the purpose, action will follow.

If you are ambiguous on your purpose – the couch will have increased utility.

Let's use training for a physical event. You know the target. You know the date. You know why you are competing. Oh wait – you do know why, right?

If your 'why' is not strong enough to overcome your 'why not' then you are not going to move.

If your clarity is compromised then it may be time to re-evaluate your choice.

If you have determined that your 'why' is strong enough then it's time to plan your 'what': you to calculate the number of days to train, the cycles that you will follow – the rest days and the nutrition required.

Very soon it will be clear if the 'why' still strong enough?

Every major situation in your life in which you will require self-discipline will follow a similar path.

This process will walk you through the evaluation process as well as the activation processes of self-control and action. It will integrate the processes so that your mind naturally adjusts to maximize the Purpose, the Clarity and the Actions required; roadblocks or conflicts will align or be removed – automatically.

And now it's time to re-enter that wonderful state of therapeutic hypnosis where changes that are important to you take place easily and effortlessly.

Take a few moments to make yourself comfortable, obviously since your eyes will be closed you are absolutely prohibited to listen to this program while operating machinery of any sort and certainly no driving – this program is very powerful and even if you do not intend to go into a state of hypnosis – do not listen to this while driving.

As you relax you notice that you are breathing in relaxation and out tension.

15

MPH Sleep now – go deeper into hypnosis than you have ever been before.

As you listen to the sound of my voice and throughout this program each breath cycle that you take, breathing in relaxation and breathing out tension takes you twice as deep twice as relaxed as you were before.

Sounds other than my voice may occur and that is fine – just allow them to be and as you hear them they will serve to double your relaxation and depth of hypnosis.

As you continue to go deeper and deeper see yourself in an amazing room filled with wonderful works of art, and as you peruse these magnificent creations you realize that each work of art is based on your life.

In one part of the room you see the idea of you – the you that existed even before you were conceived.

As you look at the sculptures of the idea of you you become twice as relaxed, twice as deep into hypnosis and that allows you to see paintings of the idea that was to become you.

Deeper and Deeper, more and more relaxed.

As you go deeper and deeper it allows you then to see you as a baby, and as you continue to progress and deepen your state of hypnosis, as a toddler.

Feel joy, feel happiness and even when life happens allow those feelings to prevail.

You continue to go deeper and deeper and you art depicting you in your youth, deeper and deeper, more and more relaxed. See the art from a variety of disciplines and enjoy the look, the feel, the emotion, the promise that is you. As you move through the gallery of art that is you you see yourself reflected in the art at each stage of your life and each stage takes you deeper and deeper, more and more relaxed.

As you are well within the therapeutic realm of hypnosis you begin to see art that appears unfinished and as you go deeper you realize that this art, art that was originated before you were an idea and is awaiting your direction before it can be completed – and this makes you happy.

You understand that you have been the artist all along and that the art that you are creating is in fact, beautiful and important.

As you listen to the sound of my voice you continue to go deeper and deeper with each word you hear.

Your focus is becoming more and more clear. Your purpose for life and your purpose for specific issues clarify instantly.

You began this program with a purpose in mind and as you consider that purpose now bring your thoughts, ideas and beliefs into alignment.

As you do this consider the conflicting ideas and beliefs that you encounter – is there any validity to them?

Does your initial purpose require modification? If so, how?

Using the instructions from the foundational hypnosis recording align all thoughts and feelings toward the appropriate purpose. Take a few moments and make this happen

1 minute music

You always make your purpose crystal clear it is time to determine your actions and the area's in which you must create results.

Your mind automatically compartmentalizes each activity – each event that requires self-discipline and this includes quality interpersonal time with your family and friends as well as with your professional, physical, spiritual and social needs, providing a perfect balance, perfect focus, perfect clarity, perfect purpose and perfect action for each one.

You choose one and only one objective to focus on at a time – you are free of anything else – nothing else exists while you complete this – you are free from anything and everything as you focus -you will complete this objective to the fullest extent possible so that everything that can and should be completed at a given time is.

Once the objective is completed your mind immediately frees itself from it so that it is completely free to give 100% focus on the next item with complete focus of purpose, clarity and action.

Once that is done you select the next highest priority to focus on and so on.

You are free.

Step by step, thoroughly, efficiently and effectively you make things happen, you enjoy making things happen, you can't wait to make things happen – your desire to do things and your ability to be clear and focused on all of the things that have to be done in order to get to the things that you want make allow you to demonstrate exactly what it means to be self-disciplined.

Your self-control is effortless because you are focused and you have passion.

You make things happen easily and effortlessly and it is always easier for you to take action after careful contemplation of all of the factors known.

Even when you rest and enjoy recreation you are able to focus on rest and recreation, being completely free of anything else.

Take a few moments and envision yourself over the next 10 years with amazing motivation. You are the one that gets things done!

You are free from distractions

You have perfect focus

You have perfect clarity

You have perfect purpose

You take any and all action with purpose & clarity

1 minute music

All internal conflicts instantly align with your purpose or are removed.

30

Experience the life that is waiting for you. The love that you have for yourself, the acceptance, the forgiveness, the humility and the confidence.

Enjoy all that your maximum self-discipline has provided.

30

I ask your subconscious to bring forward to your conscious mind anything from this session that is beneficial or life enhancing, but anything that the conscious mind is not yet ready to deal with, leave that behind until the appropriate time.

I ask your subconscious to bring you healing dreams, dreams that continue the processes you've initiated here.

And now, if it is time to sleep when I count from 1 to 5 you will ignore the instructions to return to outer awareness and you will transfer to a deep, healing, restful sleep, awakening on time and fully refreshed.

If it is time to return to outer awareness then when I count from 1 to 5 you will progressively return to a wonderful state of alert consciousness, energized, focused and motivated.

1. You have a very clear purpose

2. You have one priority and you complete that efficiently
3. You take action naturally
4. Smile you are almost there and
5. Open your eyes ready for the world.

9 THE MOUNTAIN MEDITATION

This Chapter is the Mountain Meditation for Maximum Self-Discipline

This traditional meditation helps us to develop awareness that all things change, quickly or slowly, large or small, good or bad; all things change.

It is imperative that you understand that all things change. If you are at the top you can bet that this will change. General Motors is no longer the largest corporation in the world. Sears, once the dominant retailer, has become an afterthought.

If you are at the bottom then Impermanance is your advantage – you know that all things change – you, your business, your surroundings, and your world and in that change is your opportunity.

You are older and different than you were yesterday.

Embrace Impermanance.

Take a few minutes and bring your attention to your breath, you may notice it at the tip of your nose, the cooler air flowing in and the warmer air flowing out.

15

Perhaps you notice it more in your mouth or maybe you are breathing with your belly and notice the sensations there.

30:

Bring your attention to the different parts of your body and find what works best for you. See where you are most aware of your breath.

30:

Follow through full cycles of breathing in and breathing out.

30

Feel the solid ground beneath you and you may notice a feeling of connectedness

15

Imagine that you are a mountain – you look around you and see all that takes place in your realm.

You change but very slowly, over long periods of time – but nearly everything that occurs on your domain has its own time table.

15

Look out at the wonderful Springtime. Birds are returning from their adventures beyond

Flowers are blooming

Animals that may have been hibernating are just waking up

Several species are giving birth and the new little ones are exploring their surroundings

The leaves and debris from the last fall and winter provide cover for the new growth of all kinds

30

There are storms

10

There are peaceful days

15

Temperature changes

15

The days get longer and warmer

Spend a moment with the spring

1 minute music

As time progresses the days warm, the new growth of the spring gives way to the more mature growth of the summer

15

You notice that the animals and plants are growing, maturing

15

The heat of the days warms your exposed rock often more than 100 degrees different from the other seasons

15

The sun rises and sets – the mist of the mornings, the colors of the evenings and one day becomes another

Spend a moment in the summer of your mountain

1 minute music

As the weather begins to cool, the days that began to shorten in the summer continue to do so and the beautiful colors of the fall begin to emerge.

15

The new born animals from the spring have matured, many you can't see the difference from the older ones

15

The birds begin their annual journey

The plants begin their process of preparing for the winter – creating an explosion of color

Spend a moment with the Fall

1 minute music

And as the days continue to become shorter, the nights longer the air becomes colder and one day snow appears at the top of your mountain

15

Before long snow appears lower and lower on the mountain until before long you are covered in a wonderful blanket of snow

15

The snow dampens the sounds

15

You look around and see the cycle of one day to the next and before long the days begin to lengthen again

Spend a moment with winter

1 minute music

And as the days begin to lengthen you realize as the thaw begins to take place that a whole year has passed and that spring is once again upon you.

30

Take some time with change being the object of your awareness as it relates to your Maximum Self-Discipline.

Well Done

10 THE CROSSROADS TO MAXIMUM SELF-DISCIPLINE HYPNOTHERAPY

This session is a powerful and emotional experience. If you are feeling fragile or are experiencing anxiety or depression, this is not the best time to listen to this recording.

Decisions. Commitments. Life changing events.

Being in the moment is important for experiencing life and all it has to offer.

But….

We have been given a wonderful gift of being able to imagine our future.

Our mind may be conjuring up all the things that can go wrong and distracting us from this moment, all of our exercises to date have been designed to keep this little habit at a minimum.

We may be imagining new and exciting things that we can create, new ventures, experiences, dreams and desires.

This exercise employs both of these gifts.

You are going to explore two paths in this exercise. One path is that you stay on the present course, do what you've always done, get what you've always gotten, make no significant changes and never develop Maximum Self Discipline.

One path will explore your future after you've integrated these exercises into every aspect of your being. Your future filled with Maximum Self-Discipline. Your future where important things get done, automatically. Your future in which you are in control. Your future that you fill with amazing and interesting experiences, people, opportunities and happiness. You'll create a significant emotional event and the results are quite powerful.

You decide which path is right for you.

This session is intense; if you are currently under the care of a physician or psychologist you must have them review this before you begin.

So with that thought, find a comfortable place where you can experience the wonderful world of therapeutic hypnosis, where changes that are important to you take place easily and effortlessly.

As always you are not allowed to listen to this recording when operating any type of equipment and certainly not while driving a vehicle of any sort. This will affect your outer awareness even if you do not intend to enter hypnosis at this time.

15

As you settle in begin to notice your breath. Your body is

breathing easily and effortlessly and just allow it to breathe as it needs – the wonders of the human body – you don't have to think about how much or how often to breathe at all

15

Notice that you are breathing in relaxation and breathing out tension and as you do that feel that wonderful wave of relaxation wash over you, allowing your eyes to close whenever it feels more comfortable for them to be closed rather than open.

15

MPH Sleep Now... go deeper into a state of therapeutic hypnosis than you have ever been before.

Deeper and deeper, more and more relaxed

And as you feel yourself going deeper and deeper you may from time to time hear noises other than my voice and that's fine, just allow them to be there and focus on the sound of my voice. The outside noises will just serve to relax you more and more, deeper and deeper, twice as deep with every sound.

15

Imagine if you would that you are at the top of a stair well, look around you and notice the colors, the textures, the construction.

Notice what you may be wearing – are you wearing shoes or are you bare foot?

Notice the ceiling if you would, the construction, colors, materials

Are the walls painted, wallpapered?

There are 20 stairs that we are going to walk down and as we do with each stair you'll go deeper and deeper, be more and more relaxed.

Lets go from step 20 to 19, deeper and deeper, 18 more and more relaxed, 17 safe and secure, 16 very relaxed, 15, 14 allowing your conscious mind to do whatever it needs to do, knowing that your subconscious mind will hear every word, 13, 12 deeper and deeper, 11, 10 the deeper you go the better you feel and the better you feel the deeper you go, 9, 8 wonderful, 7, 6 each breath takes you deeper and deeper throughout this process, 5, 4 sometimes you'll consciously hear me and sometimes not – and that is ok, 3, 2 and 1, very good.

The deeper you go the better you feel and the better you feel the deeper you go

It's time for your subconscious and guides to explore two paths and at the end of the exploration you will choose the path that you are to follow for the rest of your life. As you progress through this exploration you will continue to go deeper and deeper with every word that I say, with every experience that you have.

One path is to continue as you are. The concepts that are learned in this program and other are simply looked at as information and not adopted or implemented. Your life continues as it always has, regardless of the situation the results seem to always be the same. You get what you've always gotten; you've been what you've always been,

As you go out 10 years and see yourself clearly along the path that you were before you began this program. See in vivid detail like your life to come flashing before your eyes, very quickly, very vividly, very intensely.

You continue to behave without self-discipline.

Look at yourself physically is this body what you wanted?

Look at the influence that you've had on your friends and family – do you want to be responsible for the example that you set?

Is this the health that you wanted for your body?

Do you have the vitality, the energy that you wanted?

Are you physically able to do all that you wish to do or have you allowed your physical body to waste away due to not employing Maximum Self-Discipline?

Is this the mind that you wanted? Is your mind filled with wonder, curiosity, happiness, joy, curiosity, learning and teaching? If not – what is it filled with?

Does your mind get excited about new things, new hobbies,

new interests, new people, new experiences?

Does your mind have the nutrition, the physical support it needs from you – or are you allowing it to decompose prematurely because you will not employ the self-discipline required?

Look at your family and friends – is this the life that you want for them? Could you, with a clear purpose and actions have made a difference?

Experience yourself professionally – is this the life that you want for yourself? Is it fulfilling? Is it financially rewarding? Do you make a difference? Does your professional life serve its purpose?

Financially you continue as you always have. You failed to be clear as to the purpose that money, that capital had in your life and you did not take the actions required to ensure that your money, your capital worked for you. You never employed the focus the self-discipline that was in your power to enjoy the rewards that could have been yours – you let it all go!

The character flaws that you exhibited before you began this program are even more pronounced in 10 years

Your world keeps getting smaller and smaller. Fewer friends, fewer family, fewer opportunities, fewer experiences, fewer joys.

Look at how your react to people in 10 years

More and more people move away from you, there is a sense about you that keeps people away.

You don't get people and people don't get you.

You have amazing ideas but you aren't able to convey them in such a way that they are accepted.

You feel more and more left out, more certain that there is some reason that you are not getting ahead – yet more and more unwilling to take the responsibility that it is YOU that keeps you from all that you ever wanted – you are running into the same old things over and over again like being in a maze that always ends the same, because you will not employ Maximum Self-Discipline!

Go out 20 years – the same path.

You are the person that you always said you'd never be

Gone is the expectation of a better future that you had when you were young

Gone is the idealism of making the world a better place

Gone is the dream of success

Gone is so much

Take a moment and experience 20 years from now staying on the same course that you've always been on. Experience this with all of your senses, see, smell taste, fee hear all that is around you – even your 6th sense – that intuition about the world around you.

Look at what staying on that path is doing to your friends, your family your loved ones

The opportunities that never were or that were wasted

What about 30 years like this? Will you even be here and if you are – what will your state be physically, financially, personally, socially, spiritually?

60

Seeing the world in this manner is frightening – even if your life were only ordinary when it could have been extraordinary. Know that you are responsible for making this future true, know that you are responsible for making a different future true as well.

Bring yourself back to the present time now.

The previous existence has not yet happened and need never happen – you have the power to choose a different path, a different life – a life filled with excitement, adventure, success and fulfillment at every level. You have chosen a life where you exist at the highest levels of Self Discipline.

Right here, right now in this session you choose to live your life at the highest levels of Self-Discipline, immediately feel and sense changes within you; those changes affect how others react to you and those changes affect every aspect of your existence.

Immediately you experience your intense and focused concentration on the moment has been increased and continues to increase to extraordinary levels. You understand the purpose of your idea physical body and you easily and effortlessly, happily employ the self-discipline to take actions that enable your crystal clear purpose to be realized.

As you look out over the next 10 years see your physical transformation – your ideal body. You have energy and vitality; you can do anything that you want. You enjoy tremendous health. You are able to work hard and to play hard. You feel wonderful, you provide your body with everything that it needs nutritionally, through exercise, rest and sleep and it rewards you with amazing vitality and energy.

Notice the example that you set for your family and friends. See their lives transform automatically before your eyes. They need never know the other path that you may have taken.

Experience their joys, their happiness, their health, their vitality. Enjoy the amazing things that they do, knowing that your leadership, your example helped to make them possible.

Examine your Professional life with Maximum Self-Discipline over the next 10 years.

You are crystal clear as to the purpose that you have assigned to your professional life and you have employed maximum self-discipline to execute the actions required.

You have made tremendous decisions, you have taken appropriate and disciplined actions, you have made timely corrections when needed and you have created amazing success, fulfillment and joy.

Your professional achievements have provided for everything that could possibly come from your professional life.

You are a leader in your profession and your example to your family, your friends, you community, your country your world creates opportunity for all.

You have crystal clarity of the purpose that finances have in your life and you employ Maximum Self-Discipline to ensure, to guarantee that your financial resources, your capital, provides for every contingency.

Your Maximum Self-Discipline brings your physical, spiritual, financial, social, civic and family lives into perfect balance and harmony so that each accentuates the others.

Take a few moments and explore all of the other areas of your life over the next 10 years, employing Maximum Self-Discipline in each area, with perfect clarity of purpose and of action, balance and harmony. See them all come together; synergistically creating the spectacular life that you've always known was yours for the asking

30

Go out from 10 to 20 years and see the impact that your decision to employ Maximum Self Discipline at the crossroads has made

See the impact on your life and your world personally

Sense the impact on your life and your world financially

Explore the impact on your life and your world socially

Notice the impact on your world spiritually, civically

15

From twenty to 30 years, experience the impact that you've had on yourself, your friends, your family your community

You are the person that you always wanted to be, growing, developing, improving and making an impact

Notice how others experience you, you attract many interesting people

Examine the impact on your family, friends, perhaps over generations

Explore the impact on your community

This is the real you

Magnify those wonderful feelings

Take those feelings up in intensity until like the mist from a mighty waterfall it explodes forth and is absorbed by every molecule every atom that is the mist that is your body.

Make your choice – choose the life of Maximum Self-Discipline. Choose the life of health, vitality, energy and rewards of every sort, personally, financially, socially, spiritually – in every way.

10

I ask your subconscious to bring forward healing dreams that can facilitate the integration and implementation of this process. That continues the process of creating the life of Maximum Self-Discipline.

Subconscious, bring forward any recollection of any part of this process that is helpful or beneficial in any way but anything that the conscious mind is not yet ready to deal with, leave that behind to until the proper time.

If it is time for you to sleep then you will ignore my instructions to return to outer awareness and as I count from 1 to 5 you will transition into a very deep state of REM sleep, awakening on time, completely refreshed and ready for your day.

If it is time to return to outer awareness then as I count from 1 to 5 you will gradually return until I say 5 when you will open your eyes feeling wonderful in every way.

1. You employ Maximum Self-Discipline in every area of your life
2. You make the world better every day

3. Your make the people around you better every day
4. Smile you are almost there and
5. Open your eyes feeling wonderful in every way

Brian Birchmeier is a Hypnotherapist based in Flushing Michigan and the owner of Maximum Performance Hypnotherapy, LLC. His practice includes private and group hypnotherapy, business and sales coaching as well as speaking and writing.

Your input is appreciated and you may reach us at results@maxphy.com, facebook.com/maxphy or www.maxphy.com.

We hope that you've enjoyed Maximize Your Self-Discipline.